I0436831

MY JOURNEY WITH PANCREATIC CANCER

A Journey of Faith and Prayer
A Detailed Description
Of
How God and I Overcame
A Deadly Cancer Disease
And associated problems

CALVIN E. RAINS, SR.

Bloomington, IN  Milton Keynes, UK

AuthorHouse™
1663 Liberty Drive, Suite 200
Bloomington, IN 47403
www.authorhouse.com
Phone: 1-800-839-8640

AuthorHouse™ UK Ltd.
500 Avebury Boulevard
Central Milton Keynes, MK9 2BE
www.authorhouse.co.uk
Phone: 08001974150

© 2006 Calvin E. Rains, Sr.. All rights reserved.

*No part of this book may be reproduced, stored in
a retrieval system, or transmitted by any means
without the written permission of the author.*

First published by AuthorHouse 3/29/2006

ISBN: 1-4259-2424-7 (sc)

Library of Congress Control Number: 2006902300

*Printed in the United States of America
Bloomington, Indiana*

This book is printed on acid-free paper.

Acknowledgements

I first want to give thanks for the constant support of my wife Inez, our three children, their spouses, and our five granddaughters. They have all given great support and encouragement. I also acknowledge the tremendous technical and compassionate support of the medical staff at Duke University Medical Center located in Durham, North Carolina and the staff at the Ravenel Oncology and Radiation units at the Memorial Hospital in Martinsville, Virginia. Of equal importance to me were the many e-mail Prayer Partners in twelve states who supported me through this cancer treatment. The e-mail list did not dwindle, but grew week by week, as more and more people became interested in my journey. I also wish to thank the churches of Henry County and Martinsville, Virginia for their close support. All of these resources became a bridge over which God was able to give His healing power to perform a miracle of healing.

Studies by various universities and medical schools have concluded that intercessory pray can be a healing force for the sick. In the past two years three important articles have appeared in reliable magazines testifying to the healing power of prayer. My prayer partners were a great source of help to me and to my family. (Appendix A).

I am grateful also for the Internet, which has opened doors to medical information for the average citizen. This information is not a substitute for choosing a good medical center to which you trust your life. But, I have found answers on the Internet that helped me to better understand the information given to me by the medical personnel.

Of great importance and encouragement was the help Randy and Dottie Robertson in helping me to get this to a publisher so that others might be helped.

Table of Contents

Introduction

At the outset let me emphasize that I am not a medically trained person. What I have written herein is a result of my own experience and research that I have done. There may be errors in judgement. I may have reached some wrong conclusions. If you have any questions about statements I have made or conclusions I have drawn, please check with a properly trained medical professional that is trained in cancer treatment.

What I have written here is my own experience with Pancreatic Cancer. I am writing this at the end of my second year. The research I have done has been for my own understanding and for the benefit of my family. What I have written is to let the reader walk with me through the first year of my battle with this deadly form of cancer.

I am aware that every person is different, and may have different experiences. However, I know I would have benefited if I could have talked with someone who had made this journey. It is toward that end that I submit this writing.

For myself, I had never heard of Pancreatic Cancer. My first information after my diagnosis was that very few survived more than a few months with this deadly form of cancer. Needless to say, my faith was severely tested at this point. As news of my diagnosis spread among my family and friends, my Prayer Partner List began to grow. As my knowledge of my condition progressed and my understanding of the disease expanded, my faith grew stronger. It is my hope and desire that this writing will help those who may be diagnosed with Pancreatic Cancer and that their family may be comforted for their journey.

It is a frightening thing to be diagnosed with a medical problem that is almost always terminal. The majority of the information available points out that most people who have pancreatic cancer die within a few months. Statistically, only five percent of those so diagnosed live for a year or more. To be able to live for a year and to be declared cancer free is a great miracle. To still be cancer free at the end of the second year is a greater miracle. I give thanks to a Loving God.

Chapter I

THE ONSET OF
PANCREATIC CANCER

The years 2000 and 2001 were years of worldwide joy and celebration. Most of the world celebrated the year 2000 as the beginning of a new century and a new millennium. However, many saw the year 2000 as the ending of the previous century, not the beginning of a new century. I celebrated both. However, I believe the year 2001 was the beginning of a new century and a new millennium.

As the 2001 New Year began, I looked back over my life and gave thanks that I had survived 76 years of the last century. I had lived through the great depression of the thirties, served as a Navy carrier based fighter pilot in the Second World War, and as a Chaplain with the Marines in the Korean War. Now, here I was privileged to start another century and millennium. Percentage wise, few people have ever had such an opportunity. There have only been twenty-one new millenniums since the birth of Jesus Christ. . I felt this could be the best year of my life.

As the year 2001 began I was completing my fifty-fourth year as a pastor of churches. I served forty-three years as fulltime pastor of fulltime churches, three years as an active duty Navy Chaplain and eight years as Interim-Pastor for churches who did not have a pastor at the time. When my journey with cancer began I was serving a wonderful congregation.

On the fifth day of February of the year 2001 my world began to take on a new and scary picture. I began to have diarrhea and no medicine would stop it. My body began to itch all over and turned yellow. There was no breaking out, just an itch. I clawed at my body day and night. When I went to bed each night, I put a sock on each hand and arm to keep me from harming my skin in my sleep. Because of my constant activity, I moved to another bed so that I would not keep my wife awake.

On February 7, I went to my local physician. She ordered stool tests and found no bacteria. She referred me to another physician on the eighth day. On the ninth day of February this physician did an ERCP, going down my throat, to seek the cause of my discomfort. He discovered that I had a tumor on my pancreas. This tumor was blocking the discharge of bile from a duct in my pancreas. The doctor put a stint (small piece of pipe) in the duct. This stopped the itching, the jaundice and the diarrhea. He then referred me to a physician at

Duke University Medical Center, located in Durham, North Carolina.

I did not know it at first, but being referred to Duke University Medical Center was for me the very best option. On doing some research in U. S. News and World Report I discovered that Duke ranked highest in the south in treating cancer. To be treated by a medical center, which ranked higher, you would have to go to the northeast part of the country. This was out of my reach for many reasons. I also would discover that Duke University Medical Center worked closely with the cancer center in my local hospital. God was surely looking after me.

March 5, 2001, I went to Duke University Medical Center for examination. The surgeon there also did an ERCP and a biopsy. He diagnosed that the tumor was cancerous. He put a larger stint in the bile duct. He also put a "Hickman Tube" in my left chest. This is a tube into my bloodstream all the way down into my heart through which they could give me medication and later chemotherapy. The physician outlined the proposed method of treatment.

1. First, I would go to my local hospital cancer center in Martinsville, Virginia and have five (5) weeks of chemotherapy and radiation.
2. This would be followed by four (4) weeks of rest.
3. Next, I would return to Duke University Medical Center for surgery. The surgery would be the "Whipple Procedure." This would involve a removal of the cancerous part of my pancreas,

part of my stomach, two parts of my intestines, the gall bladder and then reconstruct them all back together. This surgery can take four to six hours.

4. After surgery I would spend two (2) to three (3) weeks in the hospital.

5. This would be followed by weeks of recuperation and follow-up visits

6. Then there would be four (4) months of chemotherapy administered once per week by the oncology department of my local hospital.

I was able to download information from the Internet, which supported the above form of treatment. The Internet was of great value. I could get information of any aspect of my treatment, various tubes and expectations.

Chapter II
WHAT IS PANCREATIC CANCER?

As indicated above, I did quite a bit of research on the Internet regarding pancreatic cancer. Also, as I have indicated above, I had never heard of this form of cancer before. I found out that most people only survived three to six months. I quickly discovered that the outline of treatment given me at Duke University Medical Center was the one highly recommended on the Internet: point by point.

Later in the fall, The Saturday Evening Post September/October, 2001 (pages 42-47) issue would begin a four part series on pancreatic cancer. The first issue contained pictures of the surgical procedure called the "Whipple Procedure" and extensive discussion of the disease. This procedure was developed by a Dr. Whipple beginning in 1935 and has been greatly improved over the years.

There are many web sites on the Internet that are very informative. I was able to find a list of the procedures the medical center followed.

Pancreatic cancer is, of course, cancer on the pancreas. The pancreas is a vital organ in our bodies. The two main functions of the pancreas are to create enzymes to aid digestion and to create insulin to control the blood sugar. The pancreas is spoken of as having three parts: the head, the body and the tail. If too much of the pancreas is removed the patient must wear an insulin pump as a diabetic.

I discovered that Duke University Medical Center had a lot of literature describing pancreatic cancer. There is an abundance of information on the Internet. Many of these materials will show you detailed pictures of the location of the pancreas and describe with pictures the Whipple Procedure. I am sure most medical centers qualified to perform this procedure will have an abundance of literature answering most of ones questions.

After surgery the patient will have three more tubes inserted into the stomach in addition to the Hickman tube in the chest:

a. A Feeding Tube will be placed into the small intestine. The patient will be fed through this tube until the stomach is able to take liquid food and later solid food. This is usually on the left side of the stomach.

b. Two drainage tubes will usually be placed on the right side of the stomach to allow drainage from the surgical area. It is necessary that these tubes be kept clean and usable.

It is extremely important that pancreatic cancer be treated as soon as possible. Patients who do not catch the symptoms soon enough, for whatever reason, will usually have only three to six months to live. The Saturday Evening Post article referred to above pointed out that former President Carter lost four members of his family to pancreatic cancer. At present there is no known cause of pancreatic cancer. There is some evidence that it might be genetic and thus inherited. As far as I know there was no pancreatic cancer in any of my ancestors.

It is important for all cancer patients that they not travel their journey alone. Much has been written about the healing power of intercessory prayer. (Appendix A) I discovered quickly that I did not want to travel my journey alone. Having an army of concerned people with me was of great comfort.

It also was a very special time for my wife and me to be able to share our most personal thoughts. She was always there when I cried. The chemotherapy upset my emotions and many times I could not help weeping. As a man and a combat veteran, this bothered me a great deal in the beginning. But, having a trusted friend with me helped me to deal with it. It was the sudden urge to cry that led me to resign from my church position. As time passed after completion of the chemotherapy, I would weep less. It no longer bothered me.

A cancer patient must work hard to develop and keep a positive outlook. You must not quit and you must not give up. I have been guided by an experience I had as a Navy fighter pilot flying off an aircraft carrier off the coast of Japan in WWII. On one mission I was over the Japanese Island of Shikoku, headed for a Japanese Naval Base in the water near Hiroshema. I was flying at eighteen thousand feet and at fourteen thousand feet the Japanese anti-aircraft fire was bursting and filling the sky with a black smoke and shrapnel. I had to decide what I would do. Do I quit and go home? Do I find some excuse not to dive through that deadly anti-aircraft fire? No, you just do it. I was very much afraid, but I did what I had to do.

So it was with my cancer journey, I leaned forward and did what the medical personnel told me to do, no matter how afraid I became. Don't quit! Just do what is necessary. I made myself walk on the light side of life. I sang, whistled, and laughed a lot. Sometimes stopping and lecturing myself on keeping a positive attitude. It was all the same price. Positive is more enjoyable for yourself and those around you.

Chapter III

MY REPORTS TO MY
PRAYER PARTNERS

As I began my journey with pancreatic cancer I had a number of people who wanted me to let them know of my progress. My primary method of sharing my news was by e-mail. I began with a few names of people in my area. As time passed I received other requests to be added to my reports. At the end of the first year I had seventy-two names on my e-mail list of people who were located in twelve different states. At the end of the second year the list contained almost one hundred names.

Some of them began as strangers who had heard of my journey and asked to join me. I listed them all in one group entitled, "MedReport." I received much encouragement from many of these prayer partners. Many of them said they shared my information with others. Only God knows how many people were praying for me. The responses I received were a great source of encouragement and strength for me. The following are the actual e-mail reports I sent out. This may seem like a diary, and in a sense it is. I want you to be able to walk with me through this first year of my journey. I believe that it is unnecessary for me to say that I was often afraid. Many times I asked God, "Why me Lord?" This journey even brought back memories of the fear I had in combat in WWII as a carrier based fighter pilot. Each combat mission was conducted in spite of the fear of death. This journey with pancreatic cancer began in fear that I would die.

I began to prepare my affairs to be ready. I began to bring to closure a small book that I had started a few years before: "Teach Me How to Die." This was a book for the terminally ill and their primary caregiver. This book came out of an experience while visiting a twenty-eight year old friend who was dying of AIDS. His challenge to me was, "You spend a lot of time teaching people how to live, can you teach me how to die?"

In the weeks that followed he taught me much more than I taught him. I also learned much from other dying patients who allowed me to have a close walk with them in their last days.

The following is a copy of the e-mail reports I sent to my Prayer Partners.

Phase I: Getting Ready:

February 28, 2001:

I have an appointment at Duke University Medical Center in Durham, NC. I am to go to the Clinic Building and meet with a surgeon and an oncologist to discuss my options regarding my pancreatic cancer.

March 8, 2001:

I spent four days at DUMC this week. We arrived home tonight (Thursday). Good news and bad news. I have a cancer on my pancreas. It is causing the itching and the jaundice. The doctors performed four surgical procedures. The good news is that the cancer has not spread.

I will begin chemotherapy and radiation treatments soon. It is my plan and prayer to continue at Axton Baptist Church, at least for awhile. God has delivered me many times in the past. He will do His will now.

Phase II: Radiation and Chemotherapy:

March 14, 2001:

I will begin radiation and chemotherapy next Wednesday (3/21/01). I spent two hours today getting marked for radiation. The tumor is located on the pancreas and between the two kidneys. They are trying to save the kidneys. Yesterday I spent four hours getting instructions on receiving the chemotherapy. I am all set now to begin next Wednesday with both radiation and chemotherapy. The chemotherapy will be administered by a pump, which I will wear twenty-four hours a day with fill-up once a week. Radiation will be administered once each day Monday through Friday.

All of this will last five weeks, then I go back to Duke for surgery. I will keep you posted. I appreciate the prayers and concerns.

MARCH 21, 2001:

Today (3/21/01) I began my first treatments. First, I had radiation and then was hooked up to my constant companion for the next five weeks: my computerized pump to deliver the prescribed chemotherapy. I discovered that there are different strengths of chemotherapy. I will not lose my hair. Some do with other strengths.

The pump will have a constant, twenty-four hours, seven days a week, programmed flow. The pump is carried in a small black bag hooked on a cloth belt around my waist. There is a tube coming out of the small computer pump which is attached to my "Hickman" tube which was inserted into my left breast up near my shoulder (see Chapter I, March 5, 2001). I will have to learn to sleep, bathe, dress and live with this bag around my waist for five weeks. The total bag unit measures about 4"wide, 8" long and 2"thick at its thickest point. I can unbuckle the belt and lay the bag about 5 feet away from me or hang it up in the shower. This extra tubing helps to keep the pump from getting wet in the shower. It also helps you to sleep better at night. My wife created a pocket on front of a T-shirt in which I could carry the pump at night. A great help.

The treatment team is the best I have ever had. Four nurses put their home telephone numbers on the pump instruction book with instructions to call one of them day or night if I need help. One has already called my house to check on me. I baptized her husband years ago. I am grateful for your prayers and support. May God bless you.

March 23, 2001:

I have just completed my third radiation treatment. All is going well. Yesterday they increased my radiation dose. They say there is a small chance they will get a cure with me. Before, this they told me I might have three to six months. I will reach for any ladder going up. The chemo is constant. It is in a computerized pump with canister attached. I am learning to live with it. So far, no down time. I realize I have just started, but I press on. Thanks for your concern and prayers.

March 28, 2001:

Finished my first week today. It was a little more difficult. My chemo pump ran out at 4 AM, sounding an alarm. I was fortunate to be in a medical program staffed with very compassionate nurses and doctors.

You may remember that when they gave me my computerized pump, four nurses gave me their home phone numbers with instructions to call one of them if anything went wrong. I called one of them and she met me at the hospital at 7:30 AM with a new chemo reserve.

The radiation people changed their schedule and took me for my radiation treatment, which was due at 3 PM, so I would not have to return for a second trip. Today has been a harder day, but we move on. I am so grateful for your prayers in my behalf. I do not mean to bore you with my reports, but I share with you what is happening.

APRIL 1, 2001:

Why does bad things happen to good people? God has shown us that bad things do not happen only to bad people. That is the main reason (I think) that we have the Book of Job in the Bible. He was a perfect man. God found no fault in him whatsoever, but he lost everything except his life. Maybe God sometimes lets us go through trials to show others His love, even in adversity. (Appendix C).

I think the biggest reason is that we all live in a human body in a world where it rains on the just and the unjust. If there was never darkness, we would not see the stars. If there were no valleys, there would be no mountaintops.

APRIL 4, 2001:

Today I begin my third week of a five-week course. So far things have seemed well. Blood work checked good. Platelets look ok. I have a sore on my lower lip. I am pretty tired every morning. I sleep fairly well. My sinuses stop up during the night. My nose bleeds a lot. I cannot give too much praise to the staff at the oncology and radiology departments. They go out of their way to make the way easier. They are sincere.

I am grateful for the prayers going up in my behalf. You may have noted that the Harvard University Medical School and Duke University Medical School, and others, (Reader's Digest, May 2001, Pages 109-115; Prevention Magazine, October 2002, Pages 134-139, (Appendix A) have ongoing studies to show the healing value of intercessory prayers. I know that to be true and lean on you all. God Bless.

April 10, 2001:

These last days have been more difficult. I have sores on my lips. My nose stays stopped up with clotted blood. My appetite is almost gone. I sleep a lot during the day and night. The staff at the local Ravenel Oncology Center at the Martinsville Hospital continues to do everything possible to help. The department is named for Dr. Ravenel who practiced medicine in that hospital for many years. I knew him well. The whole local unit works closely with Duke University Medical Center. My radiation doctor comes to Martinsville every week from DUMC to oversee my treatment and for others.

I had to disconnect my chemo for two days this week. I will reconnect soon. It is taking quite a bit of energy from me. But, I guess we need the chemo in the long run. Thank you for your prayers. I am not sure I could make it alone. Please know I tell the Father what you do.

APRIL 16, 2001:

I have not gotten to the "good days" yet. They are about two months away. This week has been better. They took me off chemo last week. They will decide tomorrow whether to put me back on for the remainder of the time. My mouth is better. My nose is better. I hope you had a good Easter.

APRIL 17, 2001:

Today I was placed back on my chemo pump. My mouth has cleared up and my nose and sinuses are much better. Tomorrow I will begin my last week of chemo and radiation. The last week has been a little better being off the chemo. It was the week before that was so rough. I am already feeling the chemo again. I pray it is doing its job.

If I keep on schedule after next week, I will take a four-week break and then go to DUMC for surgery. The doctor says I will be in the hospital after surgery for two or three weeks. They have some things they plan to remove. There will be recuperation after surgery. It looks like I will not be of much help for about three months. I will not give up. I will not quit. With prayer friends such as you folks, the Lord can do anything. I am going to teach my wife how to e-mail some reports while I am in the hospital. Because of my limited ability, I have resigned from Axton Baptist Church effective last

Sunday. I am not able to perform the duties expected of a pastor while going through treatment. God will repay you for the kindnesses and courage you have given to me. God Bless you each and all.

Phase III: Getting ready for surgery:

April 25, 2001:

I am a little slow getting my MedReport out because I fell asleep. It has been a hard day. I finished my chemotherapy yesterday and took my last radiation this afternoon at three o'clock. Then my wife and I went out to Axton to visit some sick people. I guess I am ok after the treatments.

I am very tired tonight. I had a funeral at eleven this morning. As it stands now, I will report to DUMC to see the surgeon on May 16. I am assuming he will do some testing to see what, if anything, the treatments did to the cancer. He has quite a number of things to remove and rearrange. He says I will be in the hospital for two to three weeks. In the meantime I have to have my "Hickman Tube" dressing changed frequently. The ladies over at the hospital will do that.

As if we did not have enough to worry about, we decided to take a nephew of Inez and his wife to the mountains. We went as far as the main highway through town only to discover the traffic stopped. My wife was driving. She stopped. Then a lady, who must have been in a great hurry and distracted, did not stop. She ploughed into the rear of our car, completely wiping out our car. The nephew and I were in the back seat. At first we could not open the rear doors. Someone outside yanked one door open and we got out.

No one was hurt badly. The niece had a scratch and an ambulance came to take her to the hospital to be checked. There were angels all around us. The young woman who was stopped in front of us and was a witness was a granddaughter of a church member and knew us. The ambulance driver reminded me I had baptized him some years ago. The State Trooper who came to investigate the accident went to school with our sons. The doctor who checked the niece at the ER reminded us I had performed his wedding a year ago.

I do not know just now what we will do about another car. We have just a little time before surgery. Have a renter now.

MAY 2, 2001:

First, thank you for praying for me. I just talked with the nurse for my surgeon at DUMC. My schedule is more clear now. I must get CT-Scans here within the next two weeks. I am scheduled to enter Duke Hospital May 21 after lunch. I am scheduled for surgery May 22. Update on my feelings: I am beginning to feel better. I still feel terrible from mid-morning to mid-afternoon. My nose is better. I think the high pollen affected my nose in a super way. Again, Thanks.

MAY 9, 2001:

Not much has changed this week. I am sending these reports to you in case you ever have the opportunity to help someone else who is going through this type of cancer. I am still having hard days. I get emotional often. I feel tired most of the time. I sleep a lot in the day. I do not like to eat. I have been off chemotherapy and radiation for two weeks. I do feel a little better each day.

Next week, May 16, I go to the Martinsville Hospital for CT-Scans. I will take these with me May 21 when I enter the hospital at Duke. I am scheduled for extensive surgery **May 22.**

The doctor says I will be in the hospital for two to three weeks (that is extensive surgery in today's medical care). I am overwhelmed by the support I am getting from people all over the area. The First Baptist Church of Collinsville made me Pastor Emeritus last Sunday. I was Pastor there for over eleven years and Interim Pastor before the present Pastor came. Everywhere I go God has placed some of His angels. I told you how many angels there were when our car was totaled. This week we had to borrow some money to buy a new car. (Insurance has not yet paid). When we went to the loan officer at the bank I told her who I was and she said, "I know who you are, you baptized me in the 1960s at FBC Collinsville." God watches over us in many ways. God Bless. Thanks for caring. You too are planting seeds, which will bring flowers along your path as He has for me.

Phase IV: Surgery:

May 21-June 4, 2001:

I entered Duke University Medical Center for surgery on May 21, 2001. Surgery was performed May 22, 2001. As I have indicated before, DUMC performs the "Whipple Procedure" for surgery. I spent two full weeks in the hospital. Most of the time I was fed through a feeding tube. Then, I was placed on a "clear liquid" diet. Finally, just before going home, I was placed on a solid food diet. I had some difficulty tolerating the many tubes placed into my body. At first I had a tube through my nose, a tube in my chest for medication, a tube in my left side for feeding and two drainage tubes in my right side.

In addition to all of these tubes, I also was on oxygen. The hospital staff took good care of cleaning all of these tubes. During my time in the hospital, I was unable to send any e-mail reports to my prayer partners. However, my wife and daughter, Ann, sent an e-mail to Prayer Partners to let them know I was ok

Phase V: Recovery from surgery:

July 22, 2001:

First report after surgery. My two weeks in the hospital were difficult. The doctors and nurses were great. I am not finished with my journey yet, but I want to take this opportunity to thank you all for the many prayers and encouragements you have given my family and to me. First, I thank each and every one of you. Some have shared my messages with others, that is great. Only God knows how many people have been praying for me. Your prayers have been a bridge over which the healing power of God could pass to me. I especially want to thank some fellows who have been a part of my life for over a half of a century. Many of my Navy Fighter Pilot friends of WWII have called and sent e-mails to encourage me. I joined this carrier-based group in the South Pacific for the last attack on Japan. These men had gone through a terrible battle at Iwo Jima where their carrier was so damaged by kamikaze planes they were forced to return to Pearl Harbor to get another carrier and then return to battle.

When I joined them they were battle experienced. I flew wing on them to try to help them do what was necessary to end the war. Now, many of them are flying wing on me to help me make a safe landing. Their support in combat and their support over the years have given me an incentive to try a little harder. Thanks guys. Lord willing I will see you next year at our reunion at Charleston, SC. So many of you have given me so much support. I thank God for you daily. I shall seek to keep you informed.

In the future I would like to try to share some of the feelings and frustrations which this cancer has brought upon my family and me. For now, thanks.

JULY 28, 2001:

Recently a very good friend made a statement that I think we all feel at times. He said he wondered why God allowed me to have cancer and why He allowed a young girl to be killed in a church bus accident recently? I can tell you there are times I too wonder why. My faith gets tested many times. In my 54 years of ministry I have momentarily wondered why many times. In Korea, as a chaplain, I stood by a young marine and watched him die. We could do nothing to save him. In WWII I saw young men die. I often wondered what they could have done in life if they had lived. I have buried many young children. Somehow we forget the essence of faith in times of stress. Let us suppose that Christians never got sick and that they were successful in all that they did. It would require no faith at all to accept Christ as savior. There are TV evangelists who present that kind of message. However, if we will just reflect for a moment we will remember that we have a relationship with God in Christ by faith, not by fact.

If you can prove something beyond the shadow of a doubt, it requires no faith to accept it. When God created mankind He gave us a free will. We are free to make choices. First, we must make a choice to give our lives into the hands of God. As a child of God we submit to His will, but we are never perfect persons in this life. We do not live in a perfect world. A believer lives as a physical person in a physical world. We drink the same water, as do unbelievers. We eat basically the same as our neighbors. We drive the same roads. We are subject to diseases and failures because that is the kind of world we live in. God does not always take away our illnesses, but He is always there to help us bear them. In my opinion, the basic reason for the Book of Job in our Bible is to address this issue. Job had everything a man might desire. God allowed Satan to take everything away from Job except his life. God knew Job's faith would survive and it did. We are not promised that we will live in this body forever. We are not promised that we will always be liked and rewarded. Look what happened to Our Lord, and He was a perfect human being. I have a lot of questions, but I also have anchors for my faith. (See Appendix B). I cannot say that I feel the presence of God all of the time. But, I have experienced His intervention enough times that "I know in whom I have believed and I stand persuaded that He is able to keep that which I have committed to Him until that day" (2 Timothy 1:12). It is much more important to know WHOM you believe than WHAT you believe. God Bless you. Your faith and prayers have given me great strength in my faith. I do not know what the future holds, but I know who holds my future and I trust Him.

August 8, 2001:

We have just returned from DUMC. Received a good report. The doctor was very pleased. He removed the feeding tube and I was very pleased. I have not used it for a month. I have been eating a regular diet. I am holding my weight (I lost 4 pounds since my last visit – a month ago) I now weigh about what I weighed when I enlisted in the Navy flight training for WWII (about

170 with clothes on). I am now down about 25 pounds below my normal weight. I do not know if I will ever gain it back. I will return to Duke next week to see the oncologist. He will tell me if I need more chemotherapy. They told me after surgery that I still had some cells that would need treatment when I was strong enough after surgery. By the way, the newest issue of the Saturday Evening Post (September/October 2001) has a special article on pancreatic cancer. This issue shows pictures of what the Whipple Surgical Procedure is like. That is what I went through. They point out that this is one of the most radical surgical procedures. I will vouch for that. I am still weak, but I am getting stronger. I do not go back to the surgeon for three months that tells you something. The doctor says that I have progressed well. I am one of the few who has some hope. Your prayers have opened the door to the Great Physician and that is why I am still alive and have hope for tomorrow. I lean forward in His name and in the strength you have given to me.

Let me brag just a little; I just received an e-mail from one of my granddaughters, who is studying at Oxford University in England this summer. What a great thing this e-mail, she was responding to my report which she received in Oxford.

SEPTEMBER 25, 2001:

I am beginning to experience great difficulty with my medical condition. My back is giving me great pain at times (most of the time). I went to see the local oncology doctor to see if he thought it was a reaction to the chemotherapy. He did not think so. He ordered an x-ray. He thought it was due to back problems. He made an appointment with a local orthopedic doctor; a friend of mine. We were able to get an immediate appointment. The orthopedic doctor said he thought I was the recipient of an aging process whereby the spine undergoes some degeneration. I have some disks in the lower part of my spine that are full of arthritis (wouldn't you know).

I find some comfort in pain pills. My diagnosis is that I have lost so much weight that my back does not have the support it once had. I am having some problems with the follow-up chemotherapy. Next week we will evaluate to see if I should continue the follow up treatments. I have some serious questions about my future. However, I am here now and I am able to see my loved ones and my friends. I enjoy each day and I plan for many tomorrows. I should not complain. I have lived an exciting life. I lived to see my five wonderful granddaughters. I have visited much of the world. I flew some of the greatest airplanes of WWII and walked beside some of the best Marines in Korea. God has delivered me over and over again. Maybe He is just bringing me in for a soft landing. I can say with Paul, "I know Whom I have believed and I am persuaded that He is able to keep that which I have committed unto Him against that day." (2 Timothy 1:12) Thanks for listening.

Phase VI: Follow-up chemotherapy:

October 3, 2001:

As I have reported, I am back on follow-up chemotherapy. I go once a week and take a shot. It acts much like it did when I took it by a computerized pump on a twenty-four hour basis for five weeks. This schedule is intended to last five months. The last few days have been increasingly worse. Yesterday was a big bad day. I had diarrhea all night and a heavy chill all morning. Inez wrapped me in blankets and I almost shook the bed apart. I ache in many places. My strength is greatly reduced. Eating is a chore. My wife works hard to provide me with something to eat, but my stomach does not want it. I have lost more weight. I now weigh about what I weighed in high school. Most of my clothes do not fit, etc. I am sorry to share so much down feelings. However, there is an up side to it all. I am now attaching a note, "My Faith Has Anchors." (Appendix B) God Bless you all.

December 19, 2001:

I am sorry that I have not updated you recently. I am in great pain. My back is in constant pain and I have not been able to sit at the computer. However, tomorrow I go to Baptist Hospital in Winston-Salem, NC for a new procedure, which I hope will relieve the pain. The best I can explain my problem is that the radiation and chemotherapy weakened the density of the backbone where the radiation went through. The doctors will not say yes or no to this.

I am to have a procedure called "vertebroplasty." The procedure is relatively new. I will lie on my stomach and these two damaged vertebrae will be filled with a cement substance, which after a period of hardening I should be able to stand without pain.

JANUARY 10, 2002:

I am having a hard time. Two vertebrae in my back have collapsed. I went to Baptist Hospital in Winston-Salem, NC and they did a procedure where they injected a "cement" to fill the cracks in the vertebrae. It was great for awhile, but soon the pain broke out in another area of my back. I can make it pretty good with a strong pain pill. The pill sends me to sleepy land sometimes. I go to DUMC next week to see if there is anything they can do. I have now lost 50 pounds and most of my energy. Because of the collapsed vertebrae in my back, I am now five inches shorter than before. I am grateful to all of you who encourage me. I draw strength and hope from you. The cold weather is getting me. I freeze all of the time and my wife burns up all the time. There is no happy medium. I let her control the heat to suit her and I put on sweaters. Please know I keep you all in my prayers. God bless you.

FEBRUARY 20, 2002:

Yesterday was my first osteoporosis visit at DUMC. The doctor was actually an endocrinologist, but he was looking after my bones. I really liked the doctor. We left home at 6:00 AM and we saw the doctor at 9:00 AM. We arrived back home around 4:00 PM. It takes us two and a half-hours driving time each way. They did a bone density test. The doctor was pleased and so was I that most of my bones showed a normal density for my age. Where the radiation went through to kill the cancer was another story. As indicated earlier, we knew two vertebrae had fractured and I had already had a procedure at Baptist Hospital. This procedure fills the space in the cracked vertebrae with cement, which is made up, in part, with ground human bones. It helps a lot, but all of the pain does not go away.

There is still arthritis and more than likely I will have some pain there for the rest of my life. One nurse told me I had a lot of old age in my back. Thanks a lot! I also saw a therapist. She showed me in great detail how to protect my bones from further damage and build some muscles. The doctor also said I needed more calcium in my diet. He did blood work and said we could get the results when we meet with the oncologist.

FEBRUARY 25, 2002:

Today we met with the surgeon who did the surgery last year and the oncologist who has guided us through all of the treatments. Last week we met with the osteoporosis doctor (endocrinologist). All three physicians reported that they find no evidence that there is any cancer in me. WOW what good news! It was a long day for us, but a good one. It is a two and a half-hour drive to the DUMC Clinic Building where we meet the doctors. We left home at 9:00 AM and we arrived back home at 9:00 PM. The doctors were overloaded and we were delayed in getting our appointments. The pain I have in my back will probably stay with me. It is possibly arthritis. They think I can control it with over-the-counter medicine. The mornings are the most difficult. Every movement from me brings a yell. It gets better as I move around. I have gained four or five pounds. Yesterday I weighed 150 pounds. I used to weigh between 190 and 198, depending of which holiday was around. I most often weighed 194 pounds; I am now shorter by 5 inches. I am working on getting my back straighter. I go back to DUMC this week to do a CT-Scan to get a closer look inside. You have helped me get good reports.

MARCH 15, 2002:

I apologize for not reporting more frequently, but there is an upside. I am doing better and there is not much new to report. We went to DUMC March 8 and had blood work and a CT-Scan. The blood work showed a vitamin D deficiency. We had not heard from the CT-Scan until last night. The oncologist called last night at 10:00 PM. He said there were no problems.

These doctors are overworked. I have felt pretty good. I still have constant pain in my back. It gets better as the day goes on. I think I can live with that. You will remember that I had two vertebrae damaged and had a procedure at Baptist Hospital. That helped, but I still have pain. Sometimes the pain is severe. I am weak, but I am able to walk a half-mile each day sometimes a full mile. I had a strange experience this week. I drove my pickup to get a new state sticker. When I sat down in the seat, I could just see over the steering wheel. Remember that I have lost 50 pounds of weight and 5 inches of height. Most of the weight came off of my rear end. I cannot sit as high in the seat. We are getting out more. I carry a pad for my back when we go to church. It protects the hump in my back. Thank you for your prayer support. I have a chance to last longer than first suggested.

MAY 2, 2002:

I apologize for the delay in this report. However, things have been changing and I wanted the latest information. Inez and I went to Charleston, SC for our biannual reunion of my WWII Fighter Pilot group. This was our first trip away from home except to see a doctor or visit the pharmacy. I made it fine. Inez drove all the way except for one hour when I drove to give her a break. The reunion went fine. We had 17 pilots present and 30 family members. We had asked each pilot to bring his children. These "children" were all adults. We all had a great time. We visited the aircraft carrier Yorktown that is a permanent memorial there. Inez and I climbed about 100 steps up to the flight deck. We both made it fine. I wanted to see the catapult on the flight deck. During the battle for Okinawa during WWII, I went to the Yorktown and flew a plane off of that carrier to take it back to my carrier.

After the reunion, we headed for DUMC in Durham, NC for a doctor's appointment for Monday. I was having some problems with my stomach. The doctor ordered a colonoscopy. I was not to eat for two days. On Wednesday I had the colonoscopy. I received a good report. As of now there is no cancer visible. My back pain is bearable. Your prayers have been used by God to create a miracle for me. Thanks.

JUNE 3, 2002:

Today we left home at 6:00 AM to go to DUMC. I saw the oncologist. He ordered a CT-Scan and blood work. The doctor said he saw no problems. I have gained 20 pounds of the 50 pounds I lost. I am still 5 inches shorter. My back still hurts. I have a knot (bow) in my spine, about midway. It still hurts if I bump it. I eat well. I walk five days per week; usually I walk a mile without stopping to rest. Some days I have to stop in the middle and rest. I am still writing books. They will probably only have a circulation among our five granddaughters. But, I will get them out of my mind. I am so grateful for your support and the blessings of God. I believe in the healing power of intercessory prayer. According to statistics, only five percent of Pancreatic Cancer patients get this far and to be cancer free at this point. God is good.

One year celebration: I sent e-mails to my surgeon and my oncologist.

To the surgeon: One year. May 22, 2001, one year ago, you performed surgery for pancreatic cancer on me.

I give thanks to God, you and your staff for this year. I feel great. I look forward to more years. Thanks.

To the oncologist: May 22 I celebrate one year of life. I want to thank you and your staff for the care and guidance you have given me. I am feeling good. I am quite active. I feel that I will go for some more years. I give thanks to God for people like you whom He can use to give me life. God bless you all

CHEMOTHERAPY AND RADIATION PERSONNEL:

I have also visited the local oncology and radiation personnel in the Cancer Center in Martinsville, VA to thank them for their help. These people were outstanding in their ability and concern.

JUNE 3, 2002:

Had an appointment with the oncologist at DUMC. He referred me to the local oncologist in Martinsville. The oncologist, the surgeon and the orthopedic doctor at DUMC have placed me on a six-month appointment schedule. Great!

SOME ACTIVITIES AFTER THE FIRST YEAR.

JUNE 9, 2002:

A fast trip to Basking Ridge, New Jersey to visit a fighter pilot friend and the Catholic Shrine of St. Joseph that had prayed for me so many times. I offered a prayer of thanksgiving in the shrine for the prayers offered in my behalf.

June 27, 2002:

Made a trip to Arkansas by way of Chicago and Memphis and driving from Memphis as far as Texarkana to visit relatives and my wife's family reunion. Made the trip fine

July 8, 2002:

Made a trip to the Northern Neck of Virginia. I had promised my wife we would go there someday. We went because July 9 was our Fifty Fifth (55) wedding anniversary. Our trip was cut short because I became sick during the night. I think I had a case of food poisoning.

Chapter IV
ASSOCIATED PROBLEM

After two of the vertebrae in my spine collapsed I had a procedure called "vertebroplasty." This involved inject-ing "cement" into my ruptured vertebrae. This would then relieve the pressure caused by the collapse. This "cement was composed in part by ground up human bones that had been removed from human bodies.

This procedure did relieve most of the pain. It did not restore my lost height. This loss in height meant that the upper rib cage was now down on, or at least close by my hipbones. This continued to cause some discomfort. This loss of upper height also affected my wearing of the suits of clothing I owned. I had to have some alterations made.

When I visited my Oncologist, he suggested I needed to see another specialist. He referred me to an orthope-dic, who in turn referred me to an endocrinologist. This last doctor felt that my testosterone was too low and that I needed to build it up. He prescribed a medication called "Androgel" for the purpose of enhancing my testosterone for the purpose of combating osteoporosis.

Throughout my battle with cancer I have always checked the Internet for a better understanding of the prescribed medication. I discovered that Androgel was primarily use for sexual enhancement. At my age of 78 years I did not feel this was what I needed. I discussed it with my wife of 55 years and we agreed that this was not proper for us.

The primary reason I felt this medication was unwise for me was the possible side effects it had. It may increase the serum cholesterol level, and it may cause an increase of the prostate.

This medication could cause prostate cancer. My father had prostate cancer and I was already fighting high cholesterol. I informed the physician that I would not take the medication.

After some back and forth communication, I finally decided I had better follow the doctor's advice. I began taking the medication.

My PSA leaped each month from 3.5 to 4.5 to 5.5 in a three-month period. The doctor wrote me to stop taking the androgel and to see a Urologist. The Urologist diagnosed me as having prostate cancer and set up a series of radiation to stop the growth.

There are three basic treatments for prostate cancer. (1) To surgically remove the prostate. (2) To implant radiated seeds. And (3) To go through radiation. The Urologist felt that for my age, and medical history that radiation was the best treatment for me and me with my history of pancreatic cancer.

I proceeded to go through thirty-seven (37) days of radiation at the Martinsville Oncology/Radiation clinic. Each day I received a radiation "shot" through each hip and front and back through my pelvic area. I had no real discomfort because of the treatment.

Within months of my radiation of my pelvic area I developed great pain. The Urologist sent me to an Orthopedic Doctor. This was the same doctor who discovered my collapsed vertebrae. He put me on a walker and began to treat me for a crack in a pelvic bone on the left side.

Using this walker greatly slowed me down as I continued to minister to my church. Getting in and out of houses I visited was difficult. When the snow came I was really at a great disadvantage. However, in time I was able to move to a walking stick and continue my work.

After three years since beginning my journey with pancreatic cancer, I am free of both the pancreatic cancer and the prostate cancer and I am still serving churches.

Chapter V

LESSONS LEARNED

EARLY DETECTION

It is vitally important with all forms of cancer to consult with your physician when you experience any symptoms out of the ordinary. This is especially important, as you grow older. As our bodies advance in years, the results of stress begin to be more apparent.

Over the years we often push ourselves to accomplish difficult tasks. Our means of employment may require us to lift heavy loads. It may require us to stand on our feet most of the day or to sit at a desk for most of the day. Generally our bodies benefit by varying our activities and exercising regularly.

When we begin to feel distress in any part of our body it often a result of over stressing that part of our body in the past.

KNOW YOUR MEDICATIONS

Each person will have a personal list of medications prescribed by the physicians who help meet their medical needs.

As we grow older we acquire new medical needs.

At the end of my first year of pancreatic cancer I could count seven different medical problems in my life. Four medical centers and now twelve different physicians monitor these needs. Each physician has a different specialty. Many extremely well qualified individual staff members of each physician and each medical facility give great healing help. Some of these I see on an infrequent basis. But, they are there if I have a need. Regular checkups are very important and usually encouraging.

I take eleven different medications on a regular daily basis. This does not count the radiation and chemotherapy, which I have taken. I have a document, which I keep current, listing the medication, its strength, frequency of taking, and the physician who prescribed it.

I have found the Internet to be of great value in understanding each illness and medication prescribed. Through this research I am better prepared to understand and treat the various side effects of medication. You know your own body's reaction better than anyone else does. You must share with your physician what your body is feeling. Much of what you share with your medical community will be of no value. But let them be the judge. Some symptoms that seem of little value to us may be warning flags to our medical personnel.

Do not quit

Various illnesses can make you a prisoner within your own body. However, only you can let outside forces make you a prisoner in you own mind. You must keep a positive attitude, no matter how negative the situation becomes.

This is especially true during the process of treatments. Radiation and chemotherapy will affect your emotions. They will drain your energy. But, you can still find ways of looking on the bright side. Almost always there is a bright side to a dark picture. Sometimes they are hard to find and difficult to maintain, but they are there.

Choose a special support person

There will be many moments during which you will need someone whom you can trust to share your frustrations and concerns. If you are married, this person will probably be your spouse. My wife and I have now been married fifty-five years. These last few years have been our best quality time. She knows the overall picture. She has been there when the medical community gave advice and cautions. As I have indicated in the early part of this writing, my wife was there to encourage right actions and to discourage wrong actions on my part.

Keep track of medical bills.

Make sure your physician and medical facility have the correct information on your health insurance. Sometimes we are treated in a state other than where we live. If you are not careful, your bills may be sent to an office in the state where treatment is given.

For instance, Blue Cross and Blue Shield (Anthem) have offices in most states. If they send your bill to the wrong state it will delay payment and may cause unnecessary worry on your part. This is especially true if you are on Medicare.

I found that it was almost impossible to match the bills with treatment dates. Some physicians and medical facilities will be billing a year later for some procedure connected with your illness. Keep a good calendar of activities and procedures.

Chapter VI

CELEBRATION OF LIFE

What a wonderful feeling and time for giving thanks for having survived pancreatic cancer and come to the end of the second year to be cancer free and almost pain free. It has been a hard journey. I have had the best medical assistance available in my area. Only God knows how many people have been praying for me. I have a feeling of thanksgiving comparable to the feeling I had during WWII when my plane crashed on the carrier, caught on fire and was hanging precariously on the side of the carrier deck. I could not get out under my own power. Two deck crewmen risked their own life to pull me out just before the plane went into the ocean. What a feeling of deliverance.

I feel sure that my battle with pancreatic cancer is not over. I still have a damaged back. I am five inches shorter. I periodically have pain in my lower back. But, I am alive and relatively active. I give thanks to God, the medical community and to my many friends for my level of health.

It is my fervent hope that God will give me opportunity to be of some encouragement to others who are forced to take the pancreatic cancer journey. That is the primary purpose for this writing. I want you to know there is hope, no matter how dark are the clouds of fear. I believe I can be of help because I have been there.

Keeping on keeping on

At this point as I write this (May 2003) I have been declared cancer free with the pancreatic cancer the second year. In the process of medical treatment of the pancreatic cancer, my prostate became cancerous. I have been treated with 37 days of radiation. May 8, 2003 I was declared to be cancer free with the prostate cancer.

Prayer

Share your concerns with others who will pray with and for you. Duke University Medical Center and Harvard Medical Center both have had articles published in Prevention Magazine and Readers Digest Magazine (See Appendix A) to say that research has proved that intercessory prayer is a healing force for the sick. Pray.

Appendix A
THE POWER OF INTERCESSORY
PRAYER

These are published articles showing that universities and medical schools have determined that prayer is a healing force.

1. Reader's Digest, May 2001, Pages 109-115 article by Linda Strohl. **"Why Doctors now believe Faith Heals because they are finding medical evidence."**

2. Prevention Magazine, October 2002, Rodale, Inc. by Ellen Michaud; Pages 134-139, **"Prayer can save your life."**

3. Roanoke Times Parade Magazine, Roanoke Virginia, March 23, 2003, by Dianne Hales, Pages 4-5, **"Why Prayer Can be Good Medicine."** " In the last 10 years, hundreds of scientific studies

– at some of the nation's top universities – have probed a link between health and religious faith. The data may surprise you."

Appendix B

MY FAITH HAS ANCHORS

Dr. Calvin E. Rains, Sr.

What sustains your faith when things continue to go badly? Most religious messages today seem to promise that if you will just have faith, everything will go well for you. You will earn more money and you will be healthy.

I believe it is true that if you put your trust in Jesus Christ things will go better in your life. But, how can your faith sustain you if your world begins to fall apart. How can you still trust when pain fills your every day?

We need a faith that is anchored in certain things that do not fade. My salvation is based in part on facts and part faith. There are some things we know as historical facts. We know that the world and universe came into being at sometime from some source. Our Evolutionist

Scientists have helped us to better understand how life and the universe evolved from one stage to another. Evolutionists deal with the **process** of evolution. They have no explanation of the **source** of the universe. I know of no **_theory_** of the source of the matter from which things evolved. Neither do they have a theory of the source of the energy that set in motion the evolutionary process, which they study.

The Bible has little to say about the **process** of change in our world. However, in the first eleven chapters of Genesis God introduces Himself to mankind as the **source** of life and all that is. When Yahweh spoke to Moses at the burning bush He gave Moses a basis for faith in God as Creator. He also introduced Moses to an explanation for the moral condition of mankind and to His plan for the redemption of mankind.

You can study the history of the human race and you will find certain constants: Mankind has always been religious. There is something within the makeup of man that tells him that there is a power outside him that in someway has some control over man's destiny.

Second, mankind has always believed in an existence beyond death. Man has often formed his own deities and explanation of existence beyond death. Mankind has always believed in good and evil. Evil persons would be punished beyond the grave and good persons would be rewarded.

NOW, from where did these concepts originate? How is it possible that for century after century the moral nature of man stayed the same? Why has there never been a perfect generation that had no poor, no wars, but only peace? If we are only natural human beings, it looks like some would have gotten it right somewhere on this globe. History records that no matter where mankind lived on the face of the world, isolated or together, he has been the same moral person.

Some believers have a problem with the story of creation as reported to Moses by God Himself. I have no problem at all. I believe the scientific explanation that it took millions of years for the world and universe, as we know it to reach its present state. You might say, "The Bible says it took only six days." That is right, I believe the Bible completely. The problem is that the six days of creation took place in eternity. They were six days of God's time. Mankind had not yet sinned. When Adam and Eve were put out of the Garden they entered the realm of time. When we die and enter into the presence of Our Lord we will enter His time, which is eternal. When Jesus comes again, time will be no more. You have time from the moment Adam and Eve sinned until Jesus comes again.

These are some of the pillars of fact that help my faith when things go bad. Believing the facts will not save you. However they serve as a window through which you can better see the Jesus of the New Testament. We are saved by faith through the grace of God. Our sins are removed by Faith in Jesus and His redeeming work on the cross. His resurrection gave proof of His life and death. Matthew 28:6 gives us a clue to how our salvation takes place. The angel told the women who were first to come to the empty tomb that Jesus was risen. The Greek for the word "risen" is an aorist passive, which means, "He has been raised." The power that brought Jesus alive from the tomb did not originate in the tomb. It did not originate in the dead body of Jesus. The power that brought Our Savior back to life again came from the throne of God. So is it with my salvation. The power to redeem me did not come from within me. It did not come from the church or from my praying friends. The power that redeemed my soul came from the throne of God where my Lord Jesus sits today.

SO, my faith is based on Scripture and is strengthened by the historical facts of the history of man. Sometimes it is hard to feel the presence of my Lord, and then I look at the world around me and remember how it all happened. I know I can trust the word of my Lord concerning what will happen from here on into eternity.

Appendix C
ADVERSITY: TEST OR OPPORTUNITY

DR. CALVIN E. RAINS, SR.

Recently I listened to a minister preach about how to handle the adversities that come into our lives. He indicated that when we come on hard times, health, financial, relationship failure, etc., we should look upon these as tests of our faith. I think they are opportunities, not tests. They do test us in many ways. However the source of the tests is not always easy to define.

First, if they are tests, then the administrator must be God who is testing our faith and obedience. I do not believe God brings adversity upon us, for any reason. Certainly adversity does come, to some more than to others. But in the Book of Job, it is not God who tests Job. It is Satan.

If God does not send these events of adversity upon us, why do they happen? I am afraid that most of the problems we face are of our own making. This does not mean that we set out to create a problem for ourselves, but through neglect or mismanagement we create a problem. This does not mean that we alone create these problems. If we are in a relationship that goes bad, there at least two persons involved making decisions. Sometimes there are circumstances beyond our individual control that creates a problem.

If we are talking about a financial crisis it may be caused by a worldwide problem. The solution may lie beyond our control. It may also come because of bad choices on our part. It may be caused from lack of proper planning.

How about a health problem that is life threatening? Some are caused by poor dietary choices. We can abuse our bodies by what we put into it. But, does that mean that if I have a life threatening health problem that it is my own fault? I do not think this is always the case. For instance, I have pancreatic cancer for which there is no cure. There is also no known cause at this time as to why this cancer comes. But, it does come for many. Some die quickly and some get some time. Actually none of us have a guarantee of tomorrow. We are all terminal.

When adversity comes I think we need to examine our own responsibility for it. Just what caused this problem for me? What could I have done to avert it? Seek advice from experts in that field. If your failure in some way helped bring this upon you, make adequate changes.

My main point in this discussion is to say that we should not look upon our problem as a test, but as an opportunity. God does not bring a test, but He is present in the opportunity. Draw closer to God. Seek His guidance. The primary concern is not the length of your life in this flesh, but the eternal existence of your soul. Having a close relationship with God can help you to find the best solution for any adversity. It will help build strong, meaningful relationships. It will help you to put the proper value on money, power, or position.

For whatever reason the adversity came, it can be an opportunity to enrich our lives. Sometimes we place the wrong values on the different aspects of our lives. When failure comes in any area of our lives where we have placed too much value, it will hit us very hard. If we have the proper value of life, we can handle the ups and downs that come.

Anytime adversity comes, for whatever reason, we should take that as an opportunity to examine our family relationships, financial situation, eating habits, etc. Time is a very precious commodity. When it is gone it cannot be redeemed. God is our refuge. We must turn to Him in good times as well as the bad times. He is better able to help us if we are on speaking terms.

About the author

Rev. Dr. Calvin E. Rains, Sr. served 58 years as a Baptist minister. He retired because he was diagnosed with Pancreatic Cancer and the chemotherapy was upsetting his emotions. He served in WWII as a Carrier based Fighter Pilot. He saw action against Japan. He was wounded once and received the Purple Heart and the Air Medal.

After WWII he became a minister. In his studies he earned four degrees from three institutions. Rev. Rains returned to active Navy Service for the Korean War as a Military Chaplain. He served various Navy Bases and served as a Chaplain with the U. S. Marines in Korea. While a military Chaplain he also served as Prison Chaplain and counselor. He also served in a Navy hospital counseling young men, who had lost arms, legs, etc. in the war in Korea to help them adjust to a new future.

He has had extensive service with HOSPICE dealing with terminally ill persons and CONTACT, a twenty-four-telephone crisis ministry.

Rev. Rains continues to minister to others who have been diagnosed as a terminal patient. He is the published author of many articles and two books, "Teach Me How to Die" for the terminally ill and "Thorn in the Flesh" a fictional account of the probable marriage of Saul of Tarsus.

www.ingramcontent.com/pod-product-compliance
Lightning Source LLC
Chambersburg PA
CBHW021250280526
45784CB00005B/2315